Tinnitus STOP!

The Complete Guide On Ringing In The Ears, Natural Tinnitus Remedies, And A Holistic System For Permanent Tinnitus Relief

Annette P. Price
Copyright© 2014 by Annette P. Price

Tinnitus STOP!

Copyright© 2014 Annette P. Price

All Rights Reserved.
Warning: The unauthorized reproduction or distribution of this copyrighted work is illegal. No part of this book may be scanned, uploaded or distributed via internet or other means, electronic or print without the author's permission. Criminal copyright infringement without monetary gain is investigated by the FBI and is punishable by up to 5 years in federal prison and a fine of $250,000. (http://www.fbi.gov/ipr/). Please purchase only authorized electronic or print editions and do not participate in or encourage the electronic piracy of copyrighted material.

Publisher: Living Plus Healthy Publishing

ISBN-13: 978-1499115086

ISBN-10: 1499115083

Disclaimer

The Publisher has strived to be as accurate and complete as possible in the creation of this book. While all attempts have been made to verify information provided in this publication, the Publisher assumes no responsibility for errors, omissions, or contrary interpretation of the subject matter herein. Any perceived slights of specific persons, peoples, or organizations are unintentional.

This book is not intended for use as a source of legal, business, accounting or financial advice. All readers are advised to seek services of competent professionals in the legal, business, accounting, and finance fields.

The information in this book is not intended or implied to be a substitute for professional medical advice, diagnosis or treatment. All content contained in this book is for general information purposes only. Always consult your healthcare provider before carrying on any health program.

Table of Contents

Introduction 3

Chapter 1: How the Ears Work 9

Chapter 2: A Close Look at Tinnitus 13

    What is Tinnitus? 13

    Different Types of Tinnitus 15

    Tinnitus Symptoms 20

    Diagnosis Procedures 21

Chapter 3: Causes of Tinnitus 27

Chapter 4: Traditional Tinnitus Treatment Options 41

Chapter 5: Treating Tinnitus with Natural Remedies 55

    Diets 55

    Nutrition 58

    Exercises 62

    Herbal Remedies 64

Homeopathic Remedies 70
Acupuncture 73
Acupressure 75
Craniosacral Therapy 76
Reflexology 76
Deep Breathing Exercises 78
Aromatherapy 78
Biofeedback 80
Neurofeedback 82
Sound Therapy 83
Color Therapy 84
Hypnotism 84

Chapter 6: Prevent Tinnitus from Returning 91

Living with Tinnitus 94

Summary 99

References 105

Introduction

Imagine that everything is right in your world...You have an incredible family, you love your job and you are the epitome of health. One day you awaken to an annoying little buzzing in your right ear. While you notice it, it doesn't impact your life too much and you don't think about it again throughout the day.

That night, as you are getting ready for bed and turning out the side lamp, the noise returns. This time something feels different. The noise is louder and feels stronger. However, you don't think too much about it as you lay your head on the pillow, feeling utterly exhausted.

As you try to relax, the noise gets louder. You turn over and lay on the alternate side of your head where the ear is experiencing the buzzing. The more you try to relax, the louder the noise becomes.

Frustrated, you turn on the television and distract yourself, finally drifting off into a restless sleep. When you wake in the morning, you feel sluggish; nonetheless you trudge out of bed and get ready for your day. You don't experience any more buzzing until that night as you turn out the side lamp and are preparing to go to sleep. The buzzing has returned. Exasperated, you again turn on the television, however this time you are unable to distract yourself from the loud noise. You try reading a book; but you are unable to concentrate.

Finally, you get out of bed and drink a glass of warm milk aware of the buzzing with every step you take. After a few hours of increasingly becoming more frustrated, you finally fall into another fitful sleep and awaken to the external buzzing of your alarm. Feeling totally exhausted, you drag yourself out of bed and prepare for a long day.

This time when you are getting ready for bed, you are aware of the buzzing in your ear. You are aware of it as you brush your teeth and wash your face. It is present as you change out of your clothes and into your pajamas.

The buzzing seems to get louder as you go through your house and turn off the lights, televisions and fans. By the time you crawl into bed, the buzzing is so loud that it feels as though your head will explode. You know you will not be able to wind down and relax enough to fall asleep so you don't even try.

You are really beginning to worry. What is going on? Suddenly the world as you know it has changed and you are beginning to spiral into a cycle of anxiety, fear and depression. You are no longer the upbeat and positive person you have always been and you are beginning to doubt yourself. Your family and friends begin questioning if you are feeling okay and your appetite is changing as you no longer feel like eating.

Since you are not sleeping, you do not have the energy to exercise. Since you are not exercising, you start to put on weight and feel even more sluggish. Not sure what else to do, and feeling slightly silly for doing so, you make an appointment with your physician and begin an ongoing regime of testing and treatments.

You may be suffering from Tinnitus. And you are not alone.

Hearing impairments affect an undetermined number of people. As the level of impairment is on a continuum, it is difficult to ascertain accurate statistics. One such hearing impairment that affects people of all ages is "ringing in the ears," or **Tinnitus**, an ailment that can range from annoying to debilitating.

Of the five senses, hearing is one of the most pronounced and one that works in conjunction with all of the others. Before we see a dog, we hear him barking or growling. Before we taste a burger, we hear it sizzle on the grill. Before we touch that cuddly kitten, we hear her purring. Before we taste that delicious desert, we hear the timer go off in the kitchen.

We learn to speak by hearing and imitating others. Soft music soothes us while loud noises may startle us. When one of our senses is not working correctly, it can throw our sense of comfort and normalcy off.

Most of us will experience Tinnitus at some point in our lives. The causes of Tinnitus vary as much as the treatments available for this condition. Additionally, the impact Tinnitus has on an individual can vary from day to day or minute to minute, depending on other factors present in that person's life.

In Chapter 2, you will learn all about different types of Tinnitus, its symptoms, and diagnosis procedures.

Tinnitus in itself is not a disease; rather it is a symptom of an underlying condition and will often require extensive testing to locate the source of discomfort. In some instances, simple lifestyle changes can minimize the inner noises or make them totally disappear. In the cases where an underlying medical condition has been determined, appropriate treatment will follow and allow the patient a reprieve from the Tinnitus.

Tinnitus can be frightening to those experiencing it. In some instances, the root cause is undetermined and as the patient experiences increasing anxiety over the situation, the Tinnitus also increases to an unbearable state. Other causes can be stress, anxiety, vascular problems, an underlying tumor, jaw problems, or even a side effect from medication. We will discuss the various causes in details in Chapter 3.

Treatment can range from changing your diet, to taking medications or undergoing surgery. You will learn about these treatment options in Chapter 4. Tinnitus patients have been subjected to a variety of clinical tests and been administered holistic and classic medical treatments.

For many patients, a combination of traditional medical and holistic treatments will assist them in finding relief. In Chapter 5 we will discuss these natural remedies and alternative treatments. Research continues to pursue treatment options and the future holds positive outcomes for the treatment of Tinnitus.

Since there is no cure for Tinnitus itself, once the symptoms cease, there is no guarantee that they will not return. However, in Chapter 6 we will discuss several ways to prevent that from happening. In addition, a combination of techniques, including exercise, relaxation, and regular medical examinations will assist the patient in managing Tinnitus upon its return.

So, are you ready for some relief from the ringing in your ears? Let's get started!

Chapter 1: How the Ears Work

To fully understand the impact of a hearing impairment such as Tinnitus, you must first understand how the ear works. According to Johns Hopkins Medicine, the ear is comprised of three main parts.

- **The Outer Ear:** The outer ear or auricle (pinna) is the part that is visible on a person. Its job is to gather sound waves and send them into the ear canal (external auditory meatus) where that sound is "amplified".

  From there, the waves move to a membrane at the end of the ear canal to the eardrum (tympanic membrane) where it vibrates.

- **The Middle Ear:** This part of the ear has the tiniest bones in the human body called the "ossicles". These are the malleus (hammer), incus (anvil) and stapes (stirrup), all of which further amplify the sounds.

Attached to an oval window connecting the middle and inner ear are the stapes. Opening to the middle ear, is the Eustachian tube. It equalizes the pressure between the air in the middle ear to the air outside the ear.

- **The Inner Ear:** When sound waves enter the inner ear, they go into the cochlea, which is filled with fluid. This fluid moves in response to the pulsations from the oval window. When the fluid (cochlea) moves, it sends 25,000 nerve endings moving. These nerve endings then transform the pulsations into electrical impulses that travel the auditory nerve to the brain, where they are interpreted into what we hear.

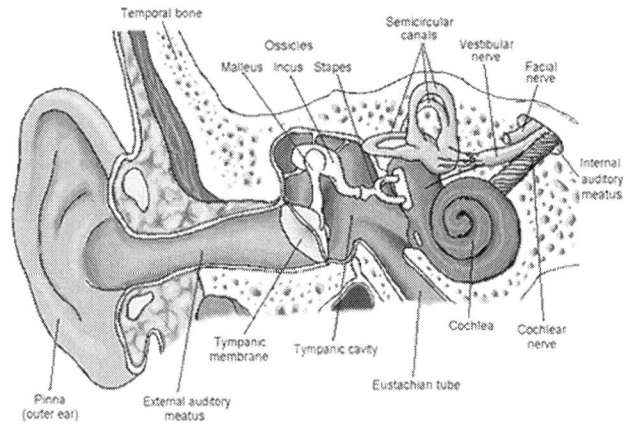

Hearing is not the ears' only job. Within the inner ear is our vestibular system, which is made up of tubes (semicircular canals) and sacs (vestibules). The American Hearing Organization teaches us that the vestibular system contains sensory receptors and is connected to the vestibular nerve that goes to the brain. This is the area in the body connected with balance, therefore when our ears are not healthy, our equilibrium may be off.

Vertigo occurs when someone's ears are not working properly and typically results from problems within the inner ear. It may be due to problems in the acoustic nerve, or disorders affecting the connections of the cerebellum and brain stem. Fluid within the ear is often a cause for vertigo symptoms and Tinnitus. Often in vertigo, one ear is healthy while the other is not, creating an inequality of balance for the patient.

Benign paroxysmal positional vertigo is the result of formation of sludge in the semicircular canals of the inner ear. This often occurs in older patients and may happen in particular positioning of the head. Vertebrobasilar insufficiency is a temporary ischemic attach that happens when the blood supply to the back of the brain and cerebellum via the arteries is reduced.

Vertigo can be debilitating for patients as it causes feelings of nausea and extreme dizziness, creating difficulty for the patient to function normally. The sense that the person is still while the world is spinning around them makes movement difficult. Often patients experience both vertigo and Tinnitus, which creates a continual feeling of unease, makes eye movements difficult, and causes the patient to continually feel off balance and nauseous.

Chapter 2: A Close Look at Tinnitus

What is Tinnitus?

The Mayo Clinic reports that Tinnitus occurs when there is a noise (buzzing, roaring, clicking, hissing or ringing) in ones' ears. While reported that Tinnitus is not in itself a disease, it is often symptomatic of other conditions requiring the patient to be further assessed by the physician. This condition may actually affect approximately 1 in 5 individuals or roughly 22 to 36 million people annually in America alone (It is difficult to obtain accurate numbers as not everyone inflicted seeks treatments).

As with other conditions, Tinnitus may present on a continuum. The symptoms may be annoying or debilitating, depending on the underlying cause and the individual patient. Tinnitus may interfere with daily activities, making it difficult for the patient to relax or sleep or even function in their normal capacity.

Hyperacusis (misophonia, phonophobia) is the over amplification of sounds in the auditory pathways. This condition arises from a variation in the central processing of sounds in the auditory pathways, eliciting an abnormal reaction from moderate sound. Patients with this condition may find low to moderate level noises disturbing and/or intolerable. While this diagnosis may occur with Tinnitus, it is not to be mistaken for Tinnitus itself.

The type of sound heard in the ears may provide an indication as to the underlying cause.

- Clicking – this could be muscle contractions in the areas around the ears. This type of sound is usually short term.

- Heartbeat – also called pulsatile Tinnitus – signifies blood vessel issues, possibly high blood pressure, an aneurysm or tumor and requires medical attention.

- Low-pitched ringing – if unilateral, this may signify Meniere's disease. It should also be noted that Tinnitus may be very loud prior to a vertigo attack.

- High-pitched ringing – typically short term and following an injury to the ear or an exposure to a loud noise. If accompanied by hearing loss, Tinnitus may become a part of the patient's life. Acoustic neuroma may also cause constant high-pitched ringing in one ear.

- Low-pitched, continuous or fluctuating noises may be the result of stiff inner ear bones (otosclerosis). Additionally, earwax, foreign particles or hairs in the ear canal rubbing against the eardrum may create different types of sounds.

Different Types of Tinnitus

Subjective Tinnitus is a condition where only the patient can hear the noise. This type of Tinnitus can occur in all three of the ear parts or it may be due to the auditory nerves or how the brain interprets the signals as sound. Some reports indicate that subjective Tinnitus begins in the inner ear when the cochleae are damaged.

Objective Tinnitus may also be known as vibratory, extrinsic or Pseudo Tinnitus. With this condition, the sound heard by the patient can also be heard by the physician or another individual within close range of the patient's ear. While objective Tinnitus is rare, it may be indicative of a blood vessel problem, inner ear issue or muscle contractions.

Pulsatile Tinnitus occurs when a patient hears his/her own heartbeat in his/her ear. Per ENT, USA, there are 4 categories of causes for Pulsatile Tinnitus:

- Arterial sounds

- Venous sounds – usually results from an increase of blood flow through the jugular vein.

- Tumor

- Spasm of the middle ear muscles – a condition where the tensor tympani muscle may contract and does not beat in sync with the heart.

For those over the age of 50, atherosclerotic coronary artery disease is often the cause of this form of Tinnitus. For individuals over the age of 60, it is normal for pressure hydrocephalus to occur. This is a slow and mild increase in the pressure of cerebral spinal fluid which eventually causes the ventricles to dilate.

Overweight females aged 20 to 50 who are experiencing pulsatile Tinnitus may be facing pseudotumor cerebri syndrome (this may also be known as idiopathic intercranial hypertension). This occurs when the pressure within the patient's skull increases, indicating an excess of cerebrospinal fluid within the skull. This condition may be the result of some medication use, such as:

- Oral contraceptives
- Trimethoprim/sulfamethoxazole
- Steroids
- Phenytoin
- Lithium
- Tetracycline
- Amiodarone
- Indomethacin

Pseudotumor cerebri syndrom may require medications or surgery to release the excess fluid within the skull. A shunt may be placed in the patient's skull to drain the fluid and help prevent it from returning. This condition may come back and the patient needs to be monitored closely by a medical professional to prevent further complications.

In addition to the different types, there are also multiple categories of Tinnitus:

- Acute Tinnitus can linger from 3 to 12 months, when it than becomes "sub-acute".

- Chronic Tinnitus inflicts patients for one year or longer and is often brought on by loud noises.

- Compensated Tinnitus is an infliction that does not interfere with patient's daily living activities.

- Chronically Complex/Uncompensated Tinnitus interferes with the patient's daily living activities and can have a severe impact on a patient's level of functioning.

Unfortunately, when some cases of Tinnitus are left untreated, they can lead to serious complications such as:

- Brain damage
- Decreased quality of life
- Trouble sleeping
- Mood disturbances
- Increased spread of cancer
- Spread of infection to other parts of the body

The prevalence of Tinnitus is difficult to ascertain as many people do not seek treatment. If the noise in the patient's ear is short term or fluctuates, the patient may just accept it without concern. When it begins to impact daily living tasks, the patient may then seek treatment from a medical professional.

Risk factors for Tinnitus as presented by the Mayo Clinic include:

- Long term exposure to loud noises.
- Caucasian.
- Male.
- Over the age of 65.
- Have age related hearing loss.
- Been diagnosed with Post-Traumatic Stress Disorder (PTSD).

The National Institute of Health reports that most disability supplement claims for Tinnitus are made by males aged 65-69 years of age. Their data shows that in self-reported cases from the mid 1990's, there was an increase of Tinnitus cases from the age of 40, with males reporting higher rates of infliction than females.

Tinnitus Symptoms

Tinnitus symptoms may be insistent or they may come and go. They give little warning of when they will begin or when they will cease. The volume of the noise level may differ from patient to patient as can the noise itself. The sounds may include ringing, hissing, clanging or thumping and they may be high pitched or low pitched. Tinnitus may make it difficult to concentrate or focus, thus impacting decision making and memory.

Symptoms that may be present with Tinnitus include:

- Headache
- Fever
- Ear pain
- A full feeling in your head

- Dizziness or Vertigo
- Fatigue
- Discharge from the inflicted ear
- Swelling of the outer ear

Additional symptoms may also be present, and may be indicative of a more serious condition. These include:

- Loss of consciousness
- Confusion
- Vertigo
- Loss of memory
- Nausea
- Bleeding

The above mentioned symptoms accompanied by Tinnitus should be treated seriously and the patient should seek immediate medical care.

Diagnosis Procedures

When a patient presents to his/her physician with a concern of Tinnitus, the physician will initially question the patient to get a better understanding of the presenting problem. Questions that may be asked include:

- When did the noises start? Have you been experiencing it for more than two weeks?

- When does it occur?

- Is it worse when you swallow?

- What does the noise sound like?

- Is it affecting your lifestyle?

- Does anything relieve the noise?

- What other symptoms are you experiencing?

- Any nausea or vomiting?

- Are you experiencing any hearing loss?

- Recent ear injuries?

- Do you experience frequent headaches?

- What medications are you currently taking? (include both prescription and over the counter medications)

- What is your alcohol use?

- What is your caffeine use?
- Do you eat fast food?
- What do you do to relax?
- Are the symptoms worse when you exercise?

The physician will likely provide an initial examination, looking into the patient's ears, eyes, nose and throat. The physician may also complete "movement" tests, in which the patient is requested to move their head and body in specific ways. This test assists the physician in identifying a potential underlying disorder if the Tinnitus is worse with any particular movements or when parts of the body are in specific positions.

Hearing screens or audiological exams will be administered to accurately assess the patient's level of hearing. This exam will also provide the physician a baseline to compare hearing screens with later exams. During this test, the patient sits in a soundproof room and wears earphones. Specific sounds will be played through the earphones and the patient will alert the technician when he/she hears the sound. This test can check whether the patient hears different ranges of sound or is having difficulty in one ear rather than both ears.

An angiography or blood vessel study may be prescribed to determine if the blood vessels are working well or are blocked. Your physician may order this test to look for underlying medical issues regarding the patient's vascular system.

A skull x-ray of the head may also be ordered. An x-ray takes pictures of the bones in the skull and allows the physician to see the patient's sinus cavities. While these pictures are not detailed they may be ordered as a starting point for the physician to diagnose the origin of a patient's Tinnitus.

Imaging tests, including a computed tomography (CT) scan of the head may be ordered. This test utilizes x-rays to show pictures of the patients head, allowing the physician to know if anything is abnormal in the patient's sinuses, brain, skull or eyes.

While the CT test is not painful, it does require the patient to lie still for a few moments while the machine circulates around the patient, creating slices, or images. Once the slices are placed together, a full picture of the patient's head is formed. A patient prepares for the test by a medical professional injecting a contrasting dye into a vein. The patient will not be able to eat or drink anything for a period of time prior to the test.

A magnetic resonance imaging scan (MRI scan) of the head may also be warranted. This test utilizes incredibly powerful magnets and radio waves to create pictures that allow the physician to see inside the patient's skull.

For the MRI scan, the patient will be required to wear no metal on their clothing nor can the patient have jewelry on. While lying on a table, the patient is slid into a scanner for approximately 60 minutes. This test may or may not require the use of contrast. If so, the dye will be given to the patient prior to the test and is provided via a vein by a medical professional. Again, the patient will not be allowed to eat or drink for an extended period of time prior to the test.

Chapter 3: Causes of Tinnitus

There is a direct correlation between being subjected to **loud noises** over a period of time and experiencing Tinnitus. Consider the musicians who are chronically exposed to loud decibel levels; after a period of time; they begin to lose their ability to hear sounds within normal ranges. Additionally, as they lose their hearing, they may experience an increase in Tinnitus.

Closed head injuries may also be a cause of Tinnitus, as the injury may directly impact the functioning of the ear. **Ear and sinus infections and neck trauma** can also be contributors to this infliction.

Some people who **continually move in specific ways or hold positions for a long period of time**, such as dancers, athletes or weight lifters may experience Tinnitus due to the strain on their neck muscles. **Cochlear de-**

terioration occurs naturally as people age and also leads to Tinnitus.

Patients who struggle with **depression, anxiety, insomnia** or other emotional impairments are also subject to the effects of Tinnitus. They may experience a decreased ability to cope with this impairment as both anxiety and depression interfere with their level of functioning in a healthy manner.

While **hearing aids** may be a treatment option for Tinnitus, they may also increase the symptoms in some patients. Close monitoring by a medical professional will assist in making the hearing aids set at a level of comfort.

Ear wax buildup and ear infections may both lead to a patient experiencing Tinnitus symptoms. By impeding the ears ability to function normally, both may exasperate the feeling of Tinnitus. Of note, any foreign body in the ear canal may also lead to Tinnitus.

Eustachian tube dysfunction from air pressure changes (airplane travel, altitude, scuba diving) or allergies may trigger Tinnitus in some patients as may spasms of the middle ear muscles.

Blood vessel disorders have been linked to this condition. **Acoustic neuroma** (tumor of the vestibulocochlear nerve) is also a common source of Tinnitus. Web MD provides the following symptoms of this disease: hearing loss, Tinnitus, headache, weakness or numbness on one side of the face, or vertigo. This typically occurs in people aged 30 to 50 and is very rare. Treatment is surgery to remove the acoustic neuroma and prevent damage to other parts of the body.

Anemia occurs when there is low iron, B12, folic acid or other nutrient levels in the body. This may occur through blood loss, damage of red blood cells, or a decrease of the body's production of red blood cells. Anemia causes weakness, skin paleness and fatigue. There is a correlation between being anemic and experiencing Tinnitus.

High blood pressure increases the blood pressure in the veins, creating excess force. This increase in energy creates other symptoms in the body, including Tinnitus. Turbulent blood flow occurs when there is narrowing or blocking in the carotid artery or jugular veins in the neck. When these conditions occur, it causes increased blood flow and leads to Tinnitus.

Labyrinthitis is inflammation of the structures in the inner ear. The cause may be viral or bacterial infections and may last days to a week. Symptoms are dizziness, vertigo and short-term hearing loss with Tinnitus. This typically goes away without medical intervention, however may respond to prescription medications if the underlying cause is bacterial infection.

Thyroid Diseases result from the thyroid not working properly. The thyroid gland is responsible for making hormones that regulate the body's energy level. Hypothyroidism occurs when the thyroid overproduces hormones while hyperthyroidism is symptomatic of the underproduction of hormones. As the thyroid is essential for energy production, it affects many different areas of the body. When it is not functioning properly, the patient may experience changes in weight, heartbeat, body temperature, muscle function and digestion. Tinnitus and vertigo may also result from thyroid dysfunction and may be regulated with medicine and/or surgery.

Food allergies may result in Tinnitus. As some people have strong reactions to specific foods, the results can be disastrous. Those allergic to grains, shellfish, milk products and eggs may have significantly increased experiences of Tinnitus when they eat these specific foods products.

TMJ (temporomandibular joint) pain is another common cause of Tinnitus as it directly relates to the functioning of the ear. Reports indicate that about 50% of TMJ sufferers are also plagued with Tinnitus. Causes of TMJ can be from stress, a jaw injury, genetics, arthritis and/or auto-immune diseases and even in ill-fitting bite. As your joint tightens and contracts, it will directly impact your hearing, sometimes contributing toward Tinnitus. Teeth grinding may also add to TMJ pain, which in turn may lead to Tinnitus.

Atherosclerosis is also a contributor to Tinnitus. As people age, cholesterol and other deposits can block the blood flow, creating an excessive force within the blood vessels. Some patients hear the pulsating beat of their heart in their ears, resulting from the pressure of increased blood flow.

AVM or arteriovenous malformation affects the connections between the arteries and veins that are near the auditory nerve. The stimulation of the pulse may result in Tinnitus. Venous sounds are those in which there is an increased blood flow in the jugular vein. This typically affects people who are pregnant, anemic or are inflicted with thyroid issues.

A **toxic reaction to medications** has been shown to cause Tinnitus. Some anti-inflammatories, antibiotics, sedatives or anti-depressants and aspirin may increase the Tinnitus. As reported in several different sites, the following types of medicines may list Tinnitus and/or hearing loss as a side effect:

- Antibiotics such as aminoglycosides, amphotericin B, chloramphenicol, minocycline, polymyxine B, sulfonamides, vancomycin.

- Antidepressants such as amitriptyline, benzodiazepines, bupropion, carbamazepine, dicofensine, doxepin, desipri-mine, fluoxetine, imipramine, lithium, melitracen, molindon, paroxetine, phenelzin, protriptilin, trazodon, zimeldin. While these medications may be prescribed for the treatment of anxiety and depression, in some patients they may also contribute to Tinnitus as a side effect.

- Antimalaria medications include chloroquine and hyroxychloroquine.

- Thalidomide.

- Aspirin Non-Steroidal Anti-inflammatory Drugs (NSAIDS) in high doses include acematacine, benorilate, benoxaprofen, carprofen, diclofenac, diflunisal, fenoprofen, feprazon or ibuprofen.

- Cancer medications, bleomycine, bromocriptine, carboplatinum, cisplatin, methotrexate, nitrogen mustard, vinblastine, vincristine. The side effects of these drugs may be decreased by monitoring the patients' blood levels.

- Diuretics such as bumetanide, ethacrynic acid, furosemide, bendroflumethazide.

- Quinine, or cloraoquine phosphate, quinacrine hydrochloride, quinine sulfate. The effects of these medications are similar to those in Aspirin products.

- Narcotic analgesics such as hydrocodone can cause Tinnitus and hearing loss.

- Mucosal Protectants such as misoprostol have been shown to contribute to hearing loss in some patients.

- Vapors or solvents such as cyclohexane, dichloromethane, hexane (gasoline), lindane, methyl-chloride, methyl-n-butyl-ketone, perchlor-ethylene, styrene, tetrachlor-ethane, toluol, and trichloroethylene.

- Anti-neoplastic medications such as bleomycin, cis-platinum, carboplatinum, methotrexate, nitrogen mustard, vinblastine.

- Cardiac Medications can be both a contributor to and a treatment for celiprolol, flecainide, lidocaine, metroprolol and procainamide.

- Sinus Medications such as quinidine and propranolol can have Tinnitus as a side effect.

- Glucocorticosteroids include prednisolone and ACTH.

- Anesthetics such as bupivacaine, tetracain and lidocaine.

- Other substances known to cause Tinnitus include: alcohol, arsenum, lead, nicotine, mercury and auronofin.

Some **auto-immune disorders** such as Lupus make it difficult for a person to fight infections and they may experience a fluid buildup in the ear canal, minimizing the ear's ability to function properly.

Lyme disease can be contracted by an infected tick and may lead to Tinnitus as Tinnitus is a side effect of Lyme.

Excess amounts of alcohol or caffeine may also lead to Tinnitus. Virtually any change in the body's chemistry could lead to difficulties in the level of ear functioning.

Environmental allergies can also be culprits as they clog the ear canals, creating a situation that leads to ear or sinus infections. Molds need very little to grow and can be devastating to individuals who are allergic to them. Pollens often trigger nasal and throat infections, leading to Tinnitus in some patients. Dust mites are virtually impossible to eliminate and can cause reactions, including nasal and throat infections.

While less thought of, household chemicals such as hairspray can also trigger allergies. As we spray our hair, the chemicals may enter into the ear canals, causing blockages, irritations or infections. Chlorinated water can also enter the ears and create inflammation which may cause further disruptions in the ear's functioning.

If the cilia (sensory cells that receive sound in the inner ear) become damaged, they may begin functioning improperly and die. Once they are damaged, they cannot be replaced. As they become damaged, they begin to create sounds that are interpreted as noise in the inner ear. Hyperactive brain cells or neurons misfiring in the brain may also cause Tinnitus.

There have been instances where Tinnitus has been brought on by lesions in the brain, near the hearing portion, or the auditory cortex. Benign tumors or meningiomas originating from brain tissue could also be significant in causing Tinnitus.

Meniere's disease is also known as Meniere's syndrome. It is named after its 1800's founder, Dr. Prosper Meniere and is a collection of symptoms with no known cause and no known cure.

Meniere's disease is an inner ear disorder that brings on dizziness and hearing loss to the inflicted patient (note that Meniere's disease does not affect the middle ear). Per report, *Classic Meniere's disease* is defined by 4 differentiating characteristics that are episodic and fluctuating:

- Episodes of rotational vertigo. Vertigo that feels to the patient like the world is "spinning." Nausea may also present, making the patient vomit. These episodes may be short in duration, giving the patient an ability to stabilize, or prolonged. The force of rotational vertigo can be on a continuum, affecting some patients mildly and others severely. Mild rotational vertigo can be compared to the "dizzies". These episodes are characterized as attacks or drop attacks and cause the patient to literally drop to the ground. The extent of time involved in these attacks also varies and can range from minutes to days.

- Episodic, low frequency hearing loss. This typically occurs in one ear rather than both. The longer the time period for this, the more extensive the hearing loss.

- Episodic Tinnitus.

- A feeling of pressure in one or both ears. While this typically occurs on just one ear, it may be present in both. The extent of fullness or pain experienced will vary from patient to patient as well as the duration.

Atypical Meniere's disease has 3 of the 4 symptoms of the classic Meniere 's disease. The following are two types of Atypical Meniere's disease.

- Cochlear hydrops with no rotational vertigo. This is a controversial diagnosis, found by some physicians to be valid while others do not recognize this condition as Meniere's disease. A cochlear hydrop occurs when there is fluid within the inner ear. As this condition directly affects hearing, it can often be misdiagnosed as a malfunction of the Eustachian tubes.

- Vestibular hydrops with no hearing loss. This is also known as vestibular Meniere's disease and again, some physicians support this diagnosis while others do not. In this atypical type of Meniere's disease, the patient has rotational vertigo, a feeling of fullness within the ear and Tinnitus, however no hearing loss is found.

Meniere's disease can inflict individuals of any age; however, research shows that most patients inflicted are between the ages of 30-50. Another characteristic of this disease is that some patients experience hyperacusis while simultaneously experiencing hearing loss. Hyperacusis and recruitment occur when a patient experiences hearing loss while becoming more sensitive to sounds.

Depression and anxiety are also common in Meniere's disease. Some patients are prone to feelings of depression and anxiety and the out of control feeling of Meniere's disease may exacerbate those issues. The inability to relax also leads some patients to be fatigued, which in turn can lead to increased levels of anxiety and stress, creating a vicious cycle of fatigue and anxiety for the patient.

Chapter 4: Traditional Tinnitus Treatment Options

Traditional medical treatment for Tinnitus has been broad and is dependent upon the results of a physician's complete examination. As one of the key indicators of Tinnitus is hearing loss, hearing aids are often prescribed. A hearing aid may be beneficial in cases where patients are experiencing sensorineural hearing loss. The hearing aid increases the sound vibrations that go into the ear where the living hair cells detect the vibrations and change them into neural signals passing them into the brain. Hearing aids can be helpful when the hearing loss is not significant.

Hearing aids are available in a choice of sizes, allowing the patients to choose one that will be a comfortable fit. Hearing aids artificially mimic the ears natural functions and are available in analog, which changes sound waves into electronic signals, or digital, which converts sound waves into numerical code. The effect of a hearing aid is contingent upon the patient being able to adjust the sound at a level that makes him/her minimize the Tinnitus.

The Mayo Clinic explains the different types of hearing aids:

- Completely in the canal – these are molded to fit inside the patient's ear canal. These are the least noticeable, less likely to pick up outside noises such as the wind, do not interfere with telephone use, and require smaller batteries, therefore requiring replacement more often than others.

- In the canal – these are custom molded and fit within part of the ear canal. They are used to improve mild to moderate hearing loss and may include features the smaller ones are unable to, such as allowing the patient to make adjustments on their own.

- Half-shell – these are smaller than the in-the-canal-hearing aid and are molded to fill the lower portion of the bowl-shaped area in the outer ear. These are used for mild to moderately severe hearing loss.

- In the ear or full shell – these hearing aids are custom made for the patient and fill most of the outer ear. These are more visible to others, are easier for the patient to insert and use larger batteries, which will require less frequent battery replacements. These can be used for people with mild to severe hearing loss.

- Behind the ear – these devices hook over the top of the ear, resting behind the ear itself. These amplify sound and carry that sound to an ear mold fit inside the ear canal. These are appropriate for all types of hearing loss.

- Open fit – these hearing aids are also behind the ear devices and are less visible to others. These are difficult for the patient to adjust and use small batteries, requiring more replacement batteries.

For hearing aids to work properly, they need to be purchased from a specialist. Be wary of buying hearing aids without the assistance of a trained professional. They can assist the new user in how to adjust the hearing aid and fit it for comfort.

The use of **wearable sound generators** allows patients who suffer from Tinnitus to wear an electronic device and essentially have "white noise" over the Tinnitus. The noise can be a multiple choice of relaxing options that will soothe the patient. "Masking" the Tinnitus takes practice and is not a quick fix for treatment.

Traditional sound generators or "white noise" machines assist the patient in relaxing and focusing on a soothing sound, thereby putting them into a position to relax. This is another form of "masking" the Tinnitus and may work well with other treatment options.

Acoustic neural stimulation is for patients with loud or chronic Tinnitus. This is similar to therapeutic biofeedback, in that the treatment desensitizes the patient to the sounds with a small electronic machine and headphones. By changing the neural circuits in the brain, the patient will learn to become less sensitized to the inner sounds.

Cochlear implants have been utilized for total hearing loss; however, for those with both Tinnitus and hearing loss, this may be an option. The implant directly stimulates the auditory nerve by going around the nonworking area of the ear. A receiver is implanted behind the ear to capture the impulses. Cochlear implants may mask the internal sounds and/or the internal sounds may be suppressed by the stimulation through the auditory nerve.

As Tinnitus is often a symptom of an underlying issue, **surgery** may be required to remove the problem. When a tumor is present, removing the tumor may provide relief for the patients' Tinnitus. When no other treatment options have been successful, a surgeon may divide the patient's auditory nerve to minimize very loud noises. Reports state that this may work 50% of the time and should be approached with caution.

Pharmacology may also be utilized in the treatment of Tinnitus. The use of anti-anxiety medications and antidepressants may be warranted when this condition has impacted the patient's quality of life. Xanax has been shown to reduce the patient's tinnitus by assisting the patient in relaxing. Prescription medications to relieve anxiety may be beneficial for patient's suffering from Tinnitus. Clonazepam at bedtime has had some success as has alprazolam with an increasing dose at bedtime as prescribed by a physician. Also, tricyclic antidepressants may be warranted to minimize the feelings of depression and anxiety that sometimes occurs in patients experiencing Tinnitus with hearing loss. Migraine medications have shown some relief as has Baclofen, which is a muscle relaxant. Gabapentin has been studied for tinnitus and while it failed to reduce the volume, it did diminish the overall force of the sounds.

Some people have found relief through the use of Lidocaine (xylocaine viscous, and zilactin-L). While this medication may provide some relief for chronic Tinnitus sufferers, it has a short term effect and is administered intravenously, making it a time consuming treatment option. Please note that this treatment may also have serious side effects and requires close monitoring by a medical provider.

TMJ treatment is imperative to those suffering from both TMJ and Tinnitus. As Tinnitus can be a result of temporomandibular joint dysfunction, when a patient treats that initial issue, the internal sounds often cease to exist. TMJ issues sometimes result from tensing the temporomandibur joint, and the patient will often hear a clicking in their ear. Treatments for TMJ include: Jaw exercises to assist the patient in relaxing and realigning the jaw joint, cranial adjustments, surgery, a change in diet to strengthen the connective tissues and a dental bite to release the tension within the joint.

Ultrasound treatments can be used for those whose Tinnitus results from sinus problems. The ultrasound locates issues within the sinuses, leading to treatment of the underlying problem. Another study has shown that inserting *Teflon plates* between the vascular loops and cochlea has shown dramatic improvement for some Tinnitus patients.

Cognitive Behavioral Therapy may also be utilized for patients also suffering from depression or anxiety. With a licensed therapist, the patient learns to distinguish between real and imagined outcomes, thus minimizing the stress level in the patient's life.

Support groups. For those patients experiencing severe Tinnitus that is interfering with their quality of life, a support group may be beneficial. Learning directly from other individuals that they are not alone in their suffering can improve a patients overall level of comfort with Tinnitus. Additionally, the patient may learn techniques for managing their

Tinnitus that they had not utilized before. For available support groups in your area, talk with your physician, counselor, or go online and search for a group you may participate in.

Overall **lifestyle changes** may be warranted for those patients suffering from Tinnitus. Decreasing stress and improving overall mood could benefit patients with low level symptoms. Increasing exercise will help to minimize stress levels and increase the patient's ability to sleep comfortably.

Caroverine Treatment

When the cochleae are not working properly, there is an excess production of glutamate and the glutamate receptors in the cochlea become overdosed with glutamate. This is known as excitotoxicity of the glutamate receptors. Glutamate is the excitatory neurotransmitter in the brain and that over production of glutamate has a toxic effect leading to cell death in the receptors. When this condition becomes chronic, it may lead to neurodegenerative diseases and possibly hearing loss and Tinnitus.

Treatment for this condition is the neuroprotective agent known as glutamate antagonist Caroverine. While this treatment has been used in Austria for years, it is not available in the United States or Canada. Caroverine is utilized by an intravenous transfusion and studies have shown that patients respond quickly. It is administered in high doses and cannot be infused over a long period of time. Other options for administering this medication are being studied, one of which allows the medication to be put directly into the ear via a transtympanic micro-catheter 2.

Tinnitus Retraining Therapy or TRT (based on the Jastreboff neurophysiological model of Tinnitus) involves retraining the patient and relearning how to function with Tinnitus. TRT utilizes psychology, psychoacoustics, physiology, neuroscience, and audiology to provide treatment for Tinnitus sufferers. Essentially, experts will retrain the patient's subconscious auditory system to accept the sounds, rather than fear them. Upon acceptance of the Tinnitus, the patient is then taught to relax the body, inhibiting the previous anxiety brought on by the Tinnitus. This is not a quick fix and will take work on the part of the patient and the professional leading the training. This method may work well in conjunction with other treatments.

TRT guidelines according to Jonathan Hazell, FRCS are as follows:

- Identify Tinnitus effect and category. The underlying issue of Tinnitus needs to be understood in order to properly treat it.

- Demystify. Learn about the Tinnitus. The more you understand the issue, the less fear it may instill.

- Get evaluated by a professional. See an Ear, Nose or Throat specialist/Audiologist for an accurate diagnosis.

- Sound enrichment. Avoid Silence! When there is no background noise, it is easy to focus primarily on the inner noise.

- Retrain your response to the Tinnitus. Be aware of your reactions when you experience Tinnitus and practice relaxation techniques to minimize your stress level.

One of the difficulties that Tinnitus sufferers experience is the inability to sleep. Some patients struggle to relax and the presence of their Tinnitus keeps them in a constant state of anxiety. Melatonin is a hormone that is secreted in the pineal gland located in the middle of the human brain. Melatonin has been shown to improve Tinnitus sufferers' sleep patterns, reducing overall anxiety and increasing the patient's ability to cope with the condition. Melatonin should not be used by pregnant or breast feeding women, patients with severe allergies or those with cancer.

Dr. Nagler, a Tinnitus expert, recommends the following guidelines for improving a Tinnitus patient's sleep:

- Use your bedroom only at night and only for sleep.

- Try to avoid naps, especially in the bedroom.

- Do not go to bed until you are sleepy; however maintain the same awaken time.

- Keep your bedroom as comfortable as possible; make it a relaxing place to be where you are surrounded by comforting objects.

- Remove the telephone or any other unwanted interruptions from the bedroom.

- If after 15-20 minutes you do not fall asleep, leave the bedroom and do something else. Do not return until you are sleepy.

- Avoid silence. Use a fan or noise machine to "mask" your Tinnitus.

According to the Jackson Ear Clinic, treatment of Meniere's disease focuses on reducing the fluid imbalance within the inner ear. Maintaining a low sodium diet and taking a diuretic may help to reduce the fluid in the endolymph (middle ear chamber). An anticholinergic medication may also be used to minimize the chemicals in the nerve endings of the inner ear in hopes of decreasing the sensitivity of those nerve endings. Medication placed under the tongue may be prescribed to combat vertigo.

As patients with Meniere's disease may cycle with their symptoms, cortisone may be used when hearing loss occurs quickly. The cortisone decreases inflammation and balances the fluid within the inner ear, working to stop the cycle.

While approximately 70% of patients with Meniere's disease respond to the above mentioned treatments, there are some who do not. Advanced treatments may be warranted and include: placement of an endolymphatic sac shunt to drain excess fluid from the ear.

An intratympanic gentamicin involves destroying the balance function to maintain the hearing. This is done to stop the vertigo and will usually stop the dizzy spells.

A vestibular nerve section cuts the balance section of the nerve to maintain the hearing section. This treatment stops alerting the brain to vertigo, thus leading to minimize the episodes.

A labyrinthectomy decreases dizzy spells, however increases the risk of hearing loss.

Chapter 5: Treating Tinnitus with Natural Remedies

Diets

When suffering from Tinnitus, it may be beneficial to increase your **potassium** and **magnesium** intake. Foods rich in these nutrients include apples, apricots, baked potatoes, leafy greens, bananas, beets and nuts. Taking a multivitamin daily may also assist the patient in obtaining nutritional values of these nutrients. Vitamin E increases the oxygen in the blood cells. Eating more whole grain, green vegetables, dried beans, fish and eggs may also minimize Tinnitus issues.

Some foods increase a patient's susceptibility to Tinnitus, such as **caffeine**, processed flours and sugars or excess animal proteins. It has also been noted that **quinine** in tonic water may directly impact Tinnitus.

The Arches Tinnitus Formula has shown some success in treating Tinnitus symptoms for various patients. The diet says to minimize the intake of salt, sugars, saturated and transfacts, nicotine, caffeine and alcohol. It has also suggests decreasing fast food and pre-packaged foods as they include high levels of sodium.

Research has shown that salt has instant effects on Tinnitus as it restricts blood vessels, thereby reducing the blood flow throughout the body. Increased levels of salt also increase blood pressure, which in turn could increase pulsatile Tinnitus.

This diet also stresses the use of **Ginkgo Biloba** and garlic in addition to the amino acid chelated zinc and bilobalide and ginkgolide B and can often be found in specific supplement form for Tinnitus sufferers.

Sugar and sugar substitutes also directly impact a patient's Tinnitus. As the brain and auditory systems have no food supply, they rely on the body's blood supply for oxygen and glucose. Research has shown that most Tinnitus sufferers are also diagnosed with hyperinsulinemia, which is a sugar metabolism disorder. Hyperinsulinemia can be a signal that a patient will eventually suffer from Type

II Diabetes. These patients may benefit from eating a diet geared for diabetics.

Sugar substitutes are also detrimental to Tinnitus sufferers. Of concern is the sugar substitute known as aspartame, or glutamate, NutraSweet, Equal and Spoonful or Indulge. Aspartame is an excitatory neurotransmitter that causes neurons to fire repeatedly until they die. This damages the nervous stems and leads to neuro-degenerative conditions.

Flavor enhancers such as MSG (monosodium glutamate) are also neuro-transmitters that trigger neurons to fire uncontrollably until they die. Of note, natural sugars in fruits and vegetables are safe and do not pose a risk for Tinnitus sufferers. Additional warning foods include: red wines, soy products, any alcohol created from grains, chocolate and avocados.

Saturated fats and trans-fats also have negative effects on the body. Saturated fats are not to be eaten by those with or at risk for diabetes. They decrease good cholesterol (HDL) while increasing bad cholesterol (LDL) and may lead to atherosclerosis. The above conditions decrease blood flow throughout the body, which can increase Tinnitus.

Unsaturated fats from nuts, vegetables and fish are healthy to eat and are prudent for the body to function properly. Unsaturated fats lower blood pressure, reduce inflammation, lower cholesterol levels and are energy sources. Omega-3 fatty acids are natural pain and inflammation reducers in addition to being mood regulators.

The **Mediterranean Diet** is also touted as safe and recommended for those suffering from Tinnitus. This diet is high in freshly prepared foods, fruits, vegetables, whole grains, beans and nuts. This diet advocates eating whole grain bread and pasta, olive oil, cheese and yogurt daily. It allows for red meat to be eaten several times per month while focusing on fish, poultry, eggs and sweets being eaten several times per week.

Nutrition

As Tinnitus can result from arteriosclerosis or high blood pressure, eating a healthy diet may reduce Tinnitus. Minimizing refined flours, sugars, and processed foods may help to lessen stress on the body and open up the arteries. Limiting animal proteins may also be beneficial.

Some people will complete a 3-day fruit and vegetable juice fast to release excess mucus in the body. Upon completion of the 3-day fast, a four-week therapy of garlic juice can be used to lower blood pressure and dilate blood vessels. This is primarily used with a vegetarian diet of whole foods and raw vegetables. It has also been shown that avoiding sugar can relieve Tinnitus by instigating an adrenalin release, which allows for vasoconstriction in the inner ear.

Vitamin B12, B6 and B5 will assist in stabilizing the inner ear fluids, therefore reducing Tinnitus. In addition to supplements, these vitamins can be found in eggs, milk, fish, poultry, lamb, oysters and yeast. Vitamin B12 is critical as it protects the nerves in the body and the ears are full of sensitive nerves, primarily the auditory nerve, whose responsibility is to send signals to the brain.

Low **magnesium** levels can cause blood vessel to constrict, including the arteries connected to the ears, causing Tinnitus in some patients. 400 mg per day of magnesium is recommended for people who are continually in a loud environment to assist in preventing the constriction. Foods to eat more of include green vegetables, whole grains, nuts and beans.

Vitamin A is imperative to have a healthy inner ear as it supports the membranes and is found in large concentrations in the cochlea. Vitamin A also is imperative for supporting sensory receptor cells throughout the body. This vitamin can be found in green leafy vegetables, blueberries, yellow fruits and vegetables or oily fish.

Vitamin D has been linked to otosclerosis, which occurs when there is an abnormal growth of bones in the ears, aggravating Tinnitus. When the patient is deficient in Vitamin D, this condition may exasperate Tinnitus symptoms and promote abnormal bone growth.

Antioxidants are imperative for preventing oxygen-caused damage to cell membranes in the body. They keep arteries open and plaque buildup free. Increasing vitamin C, vitamin E, beta-carotene and selenium can assist the body in functioning at a healthier level, minimizing the chance of Tinnitus.

Choline is known to be effective against Tinnitus when used to treat high blood pressure in some patients. Of note, this is a short term treatment.

Zinc has been utilized for older individuals who are suffering from hearing loss and Tinnitus. Zinc can be found in supplements or oysters, cereals, beans, nuts, eggs or fish. Of note, taking over 75 milligrams without medical supervision may be detrimental to the patients.

The following are the recommended daily supplements and dosages for nutritional supplements in treating Tinnitus:

- Vitamin B 12, 1 mg

- Zinc, 30 mg, with 3 mg copper

- Vitamin B complex, 50 mg twice per day

- Vitamin E, with mixed tocopherols, 400 IU

- Vitamin A, 10,000 IU (avoid during pregnancy)

Exercises

GABA (gamma-aminobutyric acid) is a neurotransmitter that inhibits electrical activity in the brain. It may reduce Tinnitus, anxiety, depression and epileptic seizures. Drs. Shulman, Arnold Strashum and Barbara Goldstien published a paper regarding the significance of GABA and its effect on Tinnitus sufferers. They wrote about a common central pathway that Tinnitus symptoms travel to get to the brain. They called this pathway, or the chemical receptor, gamma-aminobutyric acid-benzodiazepine-chloride receptor (GABA/BZ/CI) and is located in the medial temporal lobe system.

This research indicated that the function of the GABA receptor in inhibiting center nervous system synapse activity. When a patient has deficiency in the GABA receptor, it increases Tinnitus, thereby increasing anxiety and depression. This same effect can result from medications such as Neurontin and Klonopin; however it can be achieved without the side effects of the medications.

Studies have shown that exercise increases GABA levels. Participating in a one hour yoga session may increase a patient's GABA levels by over 25% without the use of medication.

Maintaining a healthy body is important in the treatment of Tinnitus symptoms. Exercise helps to keep you at a healthy weight and relieves stress. Yoga is recommended as it strengthens the body and relaxes the muscles. Additionally, exercise, specifically yoga, increases the blood flow within the body. Improving one's overall cardiovascular and cardiorespiratory health will assist in decreasing the internal sounds that create Tinnitus.

Any exercises that stimulate your overall health will improve your Tinnitus symptoms. As Tinnitus is aggravated by anxiety, decreasing your overall stress level will be imperative in alleviating your Tinnitus.

Target exercises are beneficial for the patient to focus on specific areas of the body and to relax. Dr. Murray Grossman has a specific exercise for Tinnitus sufferers as follows.

1. Standing in front of a mirror,

2. Watch your face while breathing in for 4 seconds and breathing out for 6 seconds.

3. Allow your face to relax by opening your jaw.

Do this exercise two times per week for 10 minutes. Once you have learned to relax, continue to practice for one minute per hour for 2-4 weeks until your Tinnitus has improved.

Herbal Remedies

Different sources agree on a number of herbal treatments that have been utilized in the treatment of Tinnitus.

- Ginkgo Biloba has shown to have an improvement in some cases of Tinnitus. As Gingko increases the flow of blood into the brain, it can relieve some forms of Tinnitus. This extract is obtained from a tree and is actually a combination of substances. For Tinnitus treatment, it is thought to be effective as it enhances the vascular system. It is best used for Tinnitus resulting from high cholesterol levels. This treatment has received quite a bit of attention and there is research to support both supporters and non-supporters.

- Sesame seeds have a long history with Chinese and Indian physicians in addition to herbal medicine providers for Tinnitus. These seeds may be added directly to the patient's food. Additional forms of sesame can be found in sesame candy and sesame seed spreads.

- Black cohosh has shown some relief for Tinnitus symptoms; however it is used with ginkgo.

- Zinc. There is a direct correlation between hearing loss and zinc deficiency. Eating more foods with zinc, including spinach, papaya, Brussels sprouts, cucumbers, green beans, endives, peas and prunes can increase your zinc levels. Before taking any supplement, talk with your medical provider.

- Sunflower seeds and tea made from the sunflower hulls have been long practiced in Chinese medicine to relieve Tinnitus symptoms.

- Passion flower is known for regulating neurotransmitters and helping circulate the blood flow through the body.

- Mistletoe tea also increases the blood circulation. Mix three cups of cold water and 3 tablespoons of this herb and let it sit overnight. Strain the mixture in the morning, warm and drink.

- Plantain is an extract known for maintaining healthy ears.

- Coptis and Rhubarb Combination are also known as San-huang-hsieh-hsin-tang, is utilized for hypertension related Tinnitus.

- Goldenseal has worked well in conjunction with black cohosh for some sufferers of Tinnitus. However, it is not to be used if you are pregnant or breastfeeding.

- Vinca Minor or Lesser Periwinkle has vincamine. Germans have utilized this herb for those who suffer from Meniere's syndrome and Tinnitus. Side effects form this herb include a drop in blood pressure.

- Onion Juice taken as 1 drop 3 times per week until the noise is gone, then once every 7 to ten days for maintenance. This is a folk remedy that may have little clinical support.

- Fenugreek Seed Tea may be drunk every morning, noon, and night to minimize Tinnitus.

- Ransom juice can relieve constipation which in turn may relieve Tinnitus.

- Horsetail can be taken with vegetal silica 3 – 4 times daily to reduce symptoms.

- Plantain can be drunk as juice three times daily for six weeks. The patient may also rinse ears with a plantain or calendula mixture.

- Cornus is used with yam and Chinese foxglove and mixed by an herbalist to provide positive effects for Tinnitus.

- Avena sativa comes from the wild oat plant used as a nerve tonic to help cholesterol levels, therefore increasing circulation.

- Verbena officianalis is a stress reducer that also balances the nervous system.

- Salicylic acidum is reported to provide similar results as aspirin, minus the side effects.

It is recommended to AVOID the following:

- Aspirin (in high doses) – Aspirin is a nonsteroidal anti-inflammatory drug (NSAID) used to treat fever, pain and inflammation. When used correctly, aspirin can be beneficial to the overall health of a patient. When high doses of aspirin are taken, the changes in the vascular system can lead to Tinnitus.

- Caffeine – caffeine increases blood pressure, respiration, and metabolic rate and smoothes muscles. It affects every person differently and its effects are usually felt immediately. The half-life of caffeine is typically several hours to several days, depending on the amount consumed and the size of the person. As caffeine has a direct impact on the vascular system, it can dramatically enhance a patient's Tinnitus.

- Cinchona – There is research supporting the use of this Sulphite of Quinine causing Tinnitus. Use with caution.

- Black haw – reports state that using this may aggravate Tinnitus.

- Uva ursi – can be toxic when used in high doses and known to increase Tinnitus and nausea.

- Willow bark – this may actually increase the noise of Tinnitus.

- Meadowsweet – has similar effects as aspirin and contains salicin. May increase Tinnitus.

- Wintergreen – may increase the Tinnitus noise.

- Red wine.

- Alcohol made from grains – for Tinnitus sufferers, grains are recommended to be restricted from the patient's diet.

- Marijuana use may provide some patients with relaxation benefits; however in others it may increase their Tinnitus.

Homeopathic Remedies

Homeopathic medicine originated in Germany, where it is heavily relied upon. Simplistically stated, it is based on the "law" of similia (that likes are cured by likes). The three basic principles of homeopathy are:

- Any substance may cause symptoms in a healthy person.

- Anyone with a disease has certain characteristic symptoms.

- A small amount of the substance causing symptoms in a healthy person may reduce those symptoms in a person with the corresponding disease.

The basic philosophy behind homeopathy is that homeopathic providers use diluted pills or solutions to enhance the patient's body to heal.

Homeopathic treatments can be as individual as the person using them. For Tinnitus, it is recommended that the patient takes one of the following remedies 3 times daily for two weeks, or as prescribed by a holistic practitioner:

- Salicylic acidum to relieve roaring accompanied by giddiness and hearing loss.

- Carbonium sulphuratum for roaring with a tingling feeling or if your ears are full.

- Chininum sulphuricum for buzzing or hissing.

- Kali iodatum for ringing and no other issues.

- 3X of Hydrastis every 4 to 6 hours for infection.

- 3X – 30X or Aurum for hypertension, depression, or pain.

Other homeopathic remedies include:

- Calcarea carbonica may be used for Tinnitus alone or for those experiencing vertigo.

- Carbo vegetabilis is used when Tinnitus is present with other illnesses, such as the flu and the patient is experiencing vertigo and nausea.

- China (cinchona officinalis) is for patients who also experience anxiety with their Tinnitus. It is also beneficial for fluid loss due to vomiting.

- Chininum sulphuricum may be used for buzzing, ringing and other sound to interfere with the patient's hearing.

- Cimicifuga is for patients experiencing noise sensitivity and/or pain in the neck and back.

- Coffea cruda is utilized for anxiety patients with sensitive hearing and insomnia.

- Graphites are for patients experiencing hearing loss with their Tinnitus and are also experiencing constipation.

- Kali carbonicum is used when itching and vertigo are present with the Tinnitus.

- Lycopodium is for patients experiencing hearing loss and an "echo" in their ear.

- Natrum salicylicum may be used when the Tinnitus is low key and there may also be hearing loss or vertigo. This may be used for Meniere's disease treatment.

- Salicylicum acidum is used for patients experiencing loud Tinnitus with hearing loss and vertigo. May also be used for the treatment of Meniere's disease.

Acupuncture

Acupuncture and acupressure have long been practiced for relaxation and medical benefits. Traditional Chinese medicine believes that Tinnitus is the result of a disturbance in the energy flow (chi) to the liver and kidneys. Acupuncture awakens the body's natural ability to release endorphins and promotes healing.

Acupuncturists also believe that the body is dependent on the "yin" and "yang" being balanced. Yin includes the body's blood, mucous and fluids that provide moisture and lubrication within the body. Yang represents functions such as digestion and elimination.

In acupuncture, small sterile needles are inserted into the patient's skin at specific areas. The acupuncturist has been trained to insert the needles into specific areas on the body (acupoints) to restore and reenergize the unhealthy area and restore the chi. When this occurs, the body naturally relaxes by releasing endorphins and enkephalins (natural pain relieving chemicals). This is thought to help the patient restore health and be pain free.

Acupuncture is often used in conjunction with other treatments. The patient can expect several 30 minute treatments for full healing benefits. Additional acupuncture methods may include heat, suction, friction and electromagnetic energy.

Acupressure

Acupressure was developed in Asia 5,000 years ago and has been practiced by various practitioners to ease stress, restore health and provide preventative care. Acupressure is known as shiatsu massage and utilizes touch as a healing component to reduce stress and address specific conditions and concerns.

As mentioned, ancient Chinese medicine practitioners believe that Tinnitus is a symptom of the kidney meridian being low or deficient. Stress or traumas minimize the energy flow to the kidneys, resulting in a ringing in the ears.

Per reports, the following are key pressure points to relieve Tinnitus:

- The back of the ears is a pressure point utilized to relieve headaches, anxiety and muscle neck tension. It is also beneficial in the treatment of hearing loss and Tinnitus.

- The temporal bone.

- The mastoid, behind the ears and temporal bone and slightly above the ear lobe.

- Bring your knees to your chest slowly 5 times. This exercise flattens the lower back, relieving backaches and restoring the kidneys.

- Put your finger between your belly button and pubic bone and take deep slow breaths, allowing yourself to relax for 5 – 10 minutes.

Acupressure is best utilized over a period of time and in conjunction with breathing exercises such as Yoga or Qi Gong.

Craniosacral Therapy

This therapy utilizes massage like movements to unwind the cranial and cervical bones to minimize stress and is used often in the treatment of hyperacusis. This is often used in conjunction with other therapeutic techniques.

Reflexology

Reflexology is the practice of applying pressure to the feet and hands with the clinician's thumb, finger and hand without the use of oil, cream or lotion. Based on a system of reflex areas reflecting an image of the body on the feet and hands, this therapy effects a positive physical change in the patient's body.

Reflexology utilizes techniques to improve circulation, relax the patient, and exercise the nervous system with specific pressure points. All people have pressure sensors located in the hands and feet that are related to our "fight or flight" responses. Treatment with reflexology allows for coordinating between the pressure sensors and the organs they are responsible for. A reflexology session may last from 30 – 60 minutes and upon completion, the patient should be completely relaxed.

Massage may also relieve tension, thereby minimizing Tinnitus in some patients. For example, hold the ears close to the head and use the thumbs and index fingers to massage the outer edges of both ears. The patients may also massage the area in the palm of each hand, underneath the last two fingers and/or the sole of each foot between the little and middle toe.

Toe Tensing consists of alternately relaxing and tensing your toes, which assists in alleviating the tension from the body. Do this technique while lying on your back with your eyes closed. Using your two muscles, bend toes towards you for a count of 10. Relax them and repeat 10 times.

Deep Breathing Exercises

Deep breathing exercises can be done anywhere anytime. They provide the patient the ability to take a "time out" or regroup. They also provide the patient an immediate technique to reduce stress and anxiety, allowing for refocusing.

There are many deep breathing exercise techniques. The main idea is to breathe deeply through your nostrils, and to fully extend the diaphragm. Hold for a few seconds and slowly release the air through your nostrils, feeling the diaphragm empty. Allow for time for the release of air.

Do this several times until your heartbeat slows and a feeling of relaxation comes over you.

Aromatherapy

The use of aromatherapy is not new. Smells can relax us or ignite anxiety, depending upon our experiences and likes. Specific scents have been known to help with reducing stress level, sleeping and relaxing. As the patient becomes more relaxed, they are less likely to suffer from Tinnitus.

To benefit from aromatherapy, it is suggested that you obtain some essences of your choice, dip a cotton ball into the oil and inhale deeply. These oils may also be applied directly to the skin by placing 1 to 3 drops of diluted oil into your pam and inhaling prior to placing it on the front and back of the ear lobe and the back of the neck. A vaporizer or diffuser may also be useful, when using the scents in a bedroom for relaxation.

Rosemary, cypress, lemon and rose may be used for Tinnitus when the underlying cause is blood circulation. Blending juniper, cypress and lavender can strengthen the body, relieve/reduce congestion, stimulate blood circulation, and soothe nerves. Juniper is a detoxifier and helps to expel toxins. Cypress stimulates blood circulation and relieving tension. Lavender is a decongestant and relaxant.

Peppermint and eucalyptus are known for their calming tendencies. Additional aromas may be utilized for relaxation, such as: bomeo camphor, cinnamon, cypress, garlic, onion, pine, rose, rosemary, thyme, ginger, geranium, hyssop or lemon. You may purchase the mixtures from an aromatherapist or blend them yourself by using 15 drops of each scent and putting them into a one ounce dispensing bottle.

Biofeedback

This relaxation technique teaches patients to have control over body functions, thus learning how to control their stress levels giving patients the power to influence their own automatic functions. Reducing stress has shown to have positive effects in minimizing the effects of Tinnitus.

During a biofeedback treatment, the patient is connected to sensitive electrodes. Signals are picked up from the electrodes and sent to a computer, which shows the patient's stress level by tracking body temperature, blood pressure, heart beat and brain waves.

Guiding the patient through an array of thoughts and emotions, the practitioner and patient are able to see the patient's physical reactions on the computer screen. This allows the patient to be aware of how thought/emotions directly impact his/her body and over a period of time, he/she is able to consciously control those reactions.

Biofeedback utilizes three measuring techniques: Electromyogram (EMG), temperature and galvanic skin response (GSR).

- EMG measures muscle tension when two electrodes are placed on the muscles. For Tinnitus treatment, the most common muscles impacted are the frontailis (frowning forehead muscles), the masseter (jaw muscles) and trapezium (shoulder muscles). As the machine indicates muscle tension, it gives a signal to alert the patient. The patient consciously becomes aware of the tension and begins to make the connection between feeling stress and the resulting muscle tension.

- Temperature biofeedback uses a sensor attaced to the foot or small or middle finger of the patient's dominant hand. As the patient becomes tense or anxious, the skin temperature drops due to blood being directed towards muscles and internal organs. Again, this is an effective technique in helping the patient become aware of his/her body's reactions to stimuli.

- Galvanic skin response may also be called electrodermal response (EDR). This test measures the electrical conductance in the skin, which is directly associated with the sweat glands. As the patient becomes emotionally aroused, the sweat glands become more active and the skins electrical conductivity increases.

Biofeedback treatments are typically thirty to sixty minutes and will take about 15 sessions. This is a treatment that is usually combined with other techniques.

Neurofeedback

Neurofeedback is similar to biofeedback; however it monitors a patient's brain waves. Using an electroencephalogram (EEG) with electrodes attached to a patient's forehead, electrical signals are emitted from the brain. The main brain waves are known as: Beta (awake), Alpha (relaxation), Theta (light sleep) and Delta (deep sleep).

This treatment is instrumental in teaching patients to consciously increase their alpha waves while decreasing their beta activity while working on muscle relaxation. This treatment is best utilized with other techniques.

Sound Therapy

Sound therapy has international programs enlisted to treat Tinnitus and the underlying medical reasons for the noises. These programs cause neural firing in patterns that engage different sensory and perceptive areas, including the auditory cortex, hypothalamus and limbic system, thus utilizing auditory mapping for Tinnitus sufferers.

Sound therapy utilizes hearing aid like devices, classical music, sound machines or white noise. The hope is that the external noise will "mask" the internal sounds and/or allow for auditory remapping for the patient. Of note, this treatment is done at many different levels and may differ with the professional leading the treatment. It may also be beneficial when utilized with counseling.

Color Therapy

Color therapy is a technique that uses color to balance physical, emotional, spiritual and/or mental energy. To reduce Tinnitus, use blue for thirty minutes in the morning and night, followed by 10 minutes of indigo. This therapy takes patience and symptoms will reduce over an amount of time.

Hypnotism

When a hypnotist is able to utilize hypnosis, he/she is able to relax the patient, thus relieving the patient of stress, anxiety or other concerns. The patient must be willing to let go and give the hypnotist the opportunity to relax them or this treatment will not be successful.

Per report, hypnotherapy has had positive treatment results in conjunction with other modalities. Dr. Charles Smithdeal talks extensively about the use of hypnotherapy in a written paper. He defines hypnosis as: an altered state of consciousness in which the conscious mind is temporarily bypasses, so that the subconscious mind becomes highly receptive to selective, positive suggestions. He also expands to say the following:

- Nobody may be hypnotized against their will.

- The person being hypnotized is very focused and hears every word the hypnotist says.

- The person being hypnotized will not do or say anything they do not wish to.

- The person being hypnotized will only accept and act upon positive suggestions offered for the patients benefit.

- The person being hypnotized is more in control of their mind and body under hypnosis than at any other time.

- It is not possible to become stuck in hypnosis.

To achieve maximum benefits from hypnosis, the hypnotist guides the patient to a state known as somnambulism. It is in this state that the patient becomes mentally and physically relaxed. Once relaxed, the hypnotist assists the patient in enlisting the subconscious mind to increase the control over unwanted emotions.

The patient reduces or eliminates negative thoughts and emotions regarding the Tinnitus and replaces them with positive ones. This dissipates the patient's fear of Tinnitus, thus making the Tinnitus bearable to live with.

Other Alternative Treatments include:

Chiropractic. Chiropractors believe that physical problems occur when the spine is not aligned. By applying slight pressure to different areas of the spine, these treatment providers believe they can alleviate specific physical symptoms in their patients.

Hyperbaric oxygen therapy (HBOT) has the patient breathe pure oxygen within a special chamber. The thought behind this treatment is that Tinnitus may be caused from a lack of oxygen, or a vascular issue. Having the patient breathe in pure oxygen assists the body in healthy functioning.

Low Level laser therapy is also called transmeatal irradiation therapy. Best used in the beginning of treatment and will show promise until inner hair cells die and can no longer be affected by the laser.

The **Emotional Freedom Technique** (EFT) is sometimes combined with hypnotism to defuse negative emotions quickly. EFT practices on the belief that all negative emotions stem from a disruption in the body's energy system. When a patient is consciously thinking about something that makes them uncomfortable, it generates increased energy. Positive emotions create healthy energy, negative emotions disrupt the body.

Guided Imagery is a relaxation technique that allows you to relax while you visualize yourself in a peaceful setting. While lying on your back, close your eyes. Imagine a favorite place and visualize the setting, including the sounds. Go to your favorite spot whenever you feel yourself begin to stress. This may also work prior to sleep as it helps the body and mind to relax.

Quiet Ears is a technique that has you lie on your back, relax and close your eyes. With your hands behind your head, place your thumbs in the ears and close the ear canal. You will experience a high pitched noise; focus on this sound for 5-10 minutes. This technique may help you to relax and drift off to sleep.

The Alexander Technique was invented by Frederick Matthias Alexander and encourages the physiological processes to work more efficiently and to decrease physical discomfort and stressors. Using hands, the technician releases muscular tension to improve the misalignment of the ear-bone structure.

Vibration therapy is a relatively new treatment for Tinnitus. Vibrations are used to repair the damages nerve endings in the inner ear. By using a probe, the physician places it on the mastoid bone behind the ear. A broadband sound is radiated, increasing energy to the unhealthy area. A therapy that has no scientific support is the use of Ear Canal Magnets. In this treatment, magnets are placed by the eardrums and have shown some relief for sufferers.

Wobenzym therapy utilizes enzymes to relieve Tinnitus. This treatment was originally used in the treatment of cancer; however it is now a promising treatment for Tinnitus.

In **repetitive transcranial magnetic stimulation**, electricity is passed into the brain via the scalp and skull. This is a short term treatment and is still being redefined. Additionally, when first utilized, it could bring about seizures in some patients.

Tissue salts is an additional therapy and may be utilized in the following ways:

- 12X Kali Sulph – take 3 tablets every two hours in the evening for Tinnitus night sufferers.

- Natural Mur – use 3X or 6X the potency several times per day.

- Kali phosphorica – 12X hourly until the sounds lessens, use ferrum phosphorica 6X and phosphorica 12X 3 times per day for two weeks.

- Ferr phos – 4 tablets placed under the tongue 3 times per day for Tinnitus related to blood pressure.

- Mag Phosphate – when hearing loss is involved, use 4 tablets placed under the tongue 3 times per day.

Chapter 6: Prevent Tinnitus from Returning

Most people will experience Tinnitus at some point in their life, whether due to medications, lifestyle or an underlying medical problem. Some preventative measures to reduce the probability of experiencing this condition include the following:

- Do not use cotton swabs in the ears (do not place anything into the ear as it can push wax into the ear canal).

- Wear ear plugs when necessary.

- Use headphones wisely.

- Limit exposure to excessively loud noises (gunshots, concerts).

- Practice relaxation techniques.

- Maintain a healthy lifestyle (practice nutritious eating, exercise, relax).

- Reduce caffeine and alcohol.

- Do not use tobacco products. If you currently smoke, stop (nicotine reduces blood flow).

- Maintain a healthy weight (Tinnitus often occurs more in obese people).

Consider the sounds around us and take into account that sound is measured in decibels. One decibel is one tenth of a bel, which measures the intensity of sound. For every six decibels, the intensity of sound doubles. When we reach 90dB of continued sound, the limit of us to be in that situation is 8 hours. Each time there is an increase of 6 dB, the limit of safe exposure time is reduced by half.

When talking at a whisper, we measure approximately 30 decibels. Rain falling is 50 decibels while a power saw is 110 decibels. Fireworks are about 150 decibels and a shotgun can hit 170 decibel's. When we are subjected to high levels of decibels, our ears may ring, signaling us that we need to remove ourselves from the situation or put in ear plugs.

Of course, the prevention of Tinnitus may directly relate to the underlying cause of the patient's Tinnitus. Here are some suggestions for preventing Tinnitus from recurring:

- Due to excessively loud sounds – manage your sound levels, wear ear protection

- Ear wax – maintain excellent ear hygiene.

- Anxiety and/or stress – learn relaxation techniques, exercise, remove yourself from anxiety producing situations, and talk to your physician about anti-anxiety medications.

- TMJ-jaw strengthening exercises, bite guard.

- Sinus/ear infections – talk with your physician about allergy medications.

- High blood pressure – exercise, medications.

- Vascular problems – exercise, follow a healthy diet; seek care from a medical provider.

- Thyroid – eat a healthy diet, follow medical provider recommendations.

- Medications – talk with your medical provider about alternative medications.

- Aging – exercise, relaxation techniques.

Living with Tinnitus

If, after an expanse of medical evaluations and treatments, the Tinnitus is still present, there are some things you can do. Be kind to yourself. Recognize that Tinnitus may always be a part of your life and embrace it, find ways to work with it, rather than fearing it.

Working against the Tinnitus may only make the noises louder and increase your anxiety level. As your anxiety level increases, your ability to relax decreases and this sends you into a cycle of anxiety and increased stress with minimal relaxation. This cycle is detrimental to your overall health.

Keep a diary of your triggers. Write down when your Tinnitus is better and when it is worse. This can help you figure out what your triggers are and avoid them. Consequently, this may also help you realize when your Tinnitus is better and you can begin to incorporate those foods/activities into your daily routine.

Live a healthy lifestyle. Give yourself permission to participate in activities that help you feel good. Take a class, learn a new skill or find a hobby that interests you. Exercise. Take time to walk around your neighborhood, get on the treadmill or go to the gym. Water aerobics is a good workout that is easy on the joints and can also be relaxing.

Take your medications as prescribed. Do not experiment with any medication without your doctor's approval. Some medications can have negative or toxic side effects when combined or taken in the wrong doses. Talk extensively with your provider about ALL of the medications you are taking, both prescribed and holistic.

Don't be afraid to look for additional treatments. Some treatments work better for some patients while others do not respond. Try not to get discouraged if treatments are not working. Research other options and seek out experts in those areas. Give each treatment time to work before moving onto another.

If a loved one is experiencing Tinnitus, be patient with them. This is not something they would choose to experience. Remember that they are more sensitive to noises. Fireworks or a concert may be excruciating for them. Kids yelling, dogs barking and loud singing may all trigger anxiety, which may increase their Tinnitus.

Research Tinnitus symptoms with your partner. Understand the causes and what they could mean. Prepare a list of questions to ask the physician and write down any medications that your spouse is taking. Also write down when the Tinnitus is worse and what seems to make it better.

Attend doctor's visits with your loved one. You may think of things that your loved one forgets, and having another person in attendance may provide additional support. There is a lot of information shared at a medical appointment and having you there will ensure that between the two of you, your physician's information will be heard.

Your loved one will likely need to change their lifestyle. They will need your support as they make changes in their daily living. Support their diet changes, and if possible, help them to find new recipes, assist them in cooking and eat what they eat. Go over medications together so you know what they are taking and why. Understand how each medication (prescribed or herbal) is supposed to benefit your loved one and create a schedule of when the medications are supposed to be taken.

Offer to exercise with them. Go for long walks together. Take your time and notice your surroundings, stopping often to consider your neighborhood. Take a class together or learn to do karate. Doing something together increases your relationship and will show your spouse that you are supportive of him/her.

Be patient with your loved one. As their anxiety increases, they may act differently. Give them permission to try different treatments until they find one that works for them. Attend a support group with them or help them to find a therapist.

Take over more of the household duties for a while. Remember that any additional stress on your partner may increase the Tinnitus and follow their lead with how much they can handle. Let them know how much you love them through words and actions.

Financial assistance may be available for those whose hearing may be impaired due to hearing loss and/or Tinnitus. Talk with your insurance carrier to assess what coverage is provided for you. Additionally, many states have assistive technology programs that will loan devices or finically assist them with purchasing needed devices.

Government agencies may also provide services or referrals to agencies that can assist the patient. Medicaid/Medicare may also assist with purchasing hearing aids if the patient is low income and may assist those in need and make referrals for financial assistance with medical bills.

In the United States, each state has Vocational Rehabilitation Services which may provide referrals and financial assistance for individuals of working age. United States Military Veterans may also receive reduced cost of care through the Veterans Administration. Check with local and national services to ascertain which services you qualify for to obtain assistance with evaluation and treatment.

Summary

As hearing impacts every aspect of daily life, when something interferes with this sense, it can cause stress and anxiety in a patient. Tinnitus sufferers are aware of both the physical and psychological impacts of Tinnitus. As Tinnitus in itself is not a medical condition, rather an underlying symptom of a larger medical condition, a medical exam is imperative to assess the reason for the internal noises.

As often happens, assessment and treatment takes time and the patient's anxiety increases. As the patient's anxiety increases, the Tinnitus often becomes more unbearable, thus increasing anxiety and the inability to relax. This creates a viscous cycle for the patient and may dramatically impact the patient's quality of life.

Tinnitus may be sporadic or continual. It may occur alone or by accompanied by other symptoms, such as vertigo. When it is accompanied by bleeding or severe headache, it should be examined by a medical professional immediately. Tinnitus is usually more severe at bedtime or upon first rising, when there is less outside noises and may also inhibit the patient's ability to sleep.

Tinnitus is often a symptom of an underlying disorder and there are different kinds of Tinnitus, so it is imperative to be aware of the sound, when it is most prevalent, and if there are any times the noise levels are diminished. It is vital to be honest with the medical professional so he/she can provide a thorough assessment and examination.

The patient can expect to undergo a serious of medical and diagnostic tests, including x-rays, CTs, MRIs, angiograms and/or others as warranted. Depending on the outcome of the results, the patient can expect to follow a treatment regimen to provide treatment to the underlying condition and relieve the Tinnitus.

Treatment may include medication, physical therapy or surgery. It may include one of the treatments of all of them. If the underlying cause of the Tinnitus is vascular, blood thinner medications may be warranted, if it is a tumor, surgery may be an option.

When a patient has exhausted all medical procedures and the Tinnitus continues, therapy may be an option. Learning how to relax and relieve stress is indicative in minimizing the impact that Tinnitus has on one's life. Using prescription medications to relieve anxiety and signs of depression takes time however may prove to be beneficial.

The use of alternative treatments for Tinnitus is not new. Europeans have utilized alternative techniques for centuries with positive results. Alternative therapies are exceptional ways to learn relaxation strategies, from utilizing homeopathic remedies to massage. Restoring the patient's qi through acupuncture and acupressure can provide relaxation for a patient who has been experiencing debilitating Tinnitus.

Changes in lifestyle are usually prompted, not only to relieve the Tinnitus itself, but to improve the overall functioning of the body. Following a healthier diet, reducing or minimizing caffeine and alcohol and exercising regularly will all assist the vascular system in improving blood flow. Additionally, Tinnitus typically affects individuals who are overweight and improving the lifestyle will help with weight control.

Just as there is no one cause of Tinnitus, there is no one treatment and there is no one cure. Every patient experiences Tinnitus differently and every patient responds differently to treatments. An inner noise for one person may prove to be an annoyance, however to another person it could be debilitating.

Regardless of how Tinnitus affects you, be truthful with yourself and your medical provider about how it makes you feel and what you would like to happen through treatment options. Having an open and honest conversation with your medical provider will help him/her to order the correct diagnostic tests and create a treatment plan that you are more likely to follow.

The more knowledge you have about Tinnitus, the less likely you are to fear it. Understanding the different types and what may cause them can also help you to advocate for treatments that you are comfortable with. Do not be afraid to try different treatment techniques, you may be surprised at the outcome of some. Additionally, do not be afraid to seek support for your struggles. You do not need to suffer alone. Find a support group and seek comfort from others who have experienced similar situations.

You owe it to yourself to be your own advocate. No one else understands what you are going through or how Tinnitus has impacted your life. Be proactive in your health, learn to treat yourself kindly, be forgiving of yourself and allow yourself the luxury of relaxation and kindness. Not only will you be happier, your loved ones will also benefit from the changes you are making in your life.

References

Web Sites

Abnormal Causes of Tinnitus. http://tinnituscause.com/abnormal-causes-of-tinnitus.html. Accessed 10 March 13.

Acupressure Points. http://www.acupressure.com/blog/?p=1256. Accessed 7 March 13.

Alternative Medicine for Tinnitus, http://www.holisticonline.com/Remedies/Ear/tin_alt_diet-vitamin.htm. Accessed 7 March 13.

Aromatherapy Tinnitus. http://www.aromatherapy-at-home.com/aromatherapy-Tinnitus.html. Accessed 4 March 13.

Caffeine Effects. http://www.erowid.org/chemicals/caffeine/caffeine_effects.shtml#1. Accessed 9 March 13.

Fact Sheet: Know the Power of Sound. http://www.entnet.org/HealthInformation/soundPower.cfm. Accessed 6 March 13.

Fact Sheet: How the Ears Work, http://www.entnet.org/HealthInformation/earWorks.cfm, accessed 27 February 13.

Financial Assistance: Programs and Foundations. http://www.hearingloss.org/content/financial-assistance-programs-foundations. Accessed 9 March 13.

Health & Balance, Web MD, http://www.webmd.com/balance/tc/homeopathy-topic-overview, accessed 1 May 13.

Hearing Aids. http://www.nidcd.nih.gov/health/hearing/pages/hearingaid.aspx. Accessed 3 May 13.

Hazell, Johathan, FRCS. Tinnitus Retraining Therapy: guidelines and exercises for patients.

http://www.Tinnitus.org/home/frame/guidelines.htm. Accessed 3 August 13.

Hypnotherapy and Tinnitus. http://www.Tinnitusformula.com/library/hypnotherapy-and-Tinnitus/. Accessed 4 March 13.

Kohn, Beth, Acupuncture and Tinnitus. http://www.Tinnitusformula.com/library/acupuncture-and-Tinnitus/. Accessed 4 August 13.

Hearing and Balance Center, How Normal Ear Works, http://www.umm.edu/otolaryngology/ear_works.htm, accessed 27 February 13.

Hearing Disorders and Deafness, http://www.nlm.nih.gov/medlineplus/hearingdisordersanddeafness.html, accessed 28 August 13.

How the Ear Works, http://www.hopkinsmedicine.org/hearing/hearing_loss/how_the_ear_works.html, accessed 27 July 13.

Keate, Barry. How Yoga Increases GABA and Improves Tinnitus. http://www.Tinnitusformula.com/library/how-yoga-increases-gaba-and-improves-Tinnitus/. Accessed 4 March 13.

Ototoxic Medications, Drugs that can cause hearing loss and tinnitus. League for the Hard of Hearing. http://www.chchearing.org/. Accessed 9 March 13.

Pray, J, Pray, S. Tinnitus: When the Ears Ring, US Pharmacist, 2005; 30(6). http://www.medscape.com/viewarticle/506920. Accessed 29 February 13.

Prevalence of Chronic Tinnitus, http://www.nidcd.nih.gov/health/statistics/Pages/prevalence.aspx, accessed 28 June 13.

Pulsatile Tinnitus, http://www.entusa.com/pulsatile_Tinnitus.htm. Accessed 3 May 13.

Silencing the Ring. http://library.mothernature.com/l/preventions-healing-with-vitamins/tinnitus_1018.html. Accessed 8 May 13.

Statistics about Hearing, Balance, Ear Infections, and Deafness, http://www.nidcd.nih.gov/health/statistics/pages/hearing.aspx, accessed 28 July 13,

Symptoms of Meniere's Disease, http://www.menieresinfo.com/symptoms.html#menieres-disease-is, accessed 29 July 13.

Tinnitus, http://www.sinuswars.com/tinnitus/index.asp. Accessed 8, May 13.

Tinnitus info center in holisticonline.com. http://www.holisticonline.com/remedies/ear/tin_home.htm, accessed 1 March 13.

Tinnitus, http://www.merckmanuals.com/professional/ear_nose_and_throat_disorders/approach_to_the_patient_with_ear_problems/Tinnitus.html. Accessed 2 August 13.

The Tinnitus and Hyperacusis Centre, London UK - http://www.Tinnitus.org/home/frame/THC1.htm, accessed 1 May 13.

Tinnitus, http://www.t-gone.com/. Accessed 4 March 13.

Tinnitus, http://www.nidcd.nih.gov/health/hearing/Pages/Tinnitus.aspx#1, accessed 29 February 13.

Tinnitus What is it, http://Tinnituswhatisit.com/Tinnitus-hypnotherapy-hypnotism-as-alternative-therapy/, accessed 1 March 13.

Tinnitus Review. http://www.Tinnitusreview.com/. Accessed 7 March, 13.

Tinnitus Treatments: Which ones have you tried? http://thebuzzstopshear.com/2012/02/Tinnitus-treatments-which-ones-have-you-tried/. Accessed 3 March, 13.

TMD (TMJ Jaw Joint Disorder). http://Tinnitus-free.com/Tinnitus-cures-and-causes/tmd-tmj-jaw-joint-disorder/. Accessed 3 August 13.

Top 17 Tinnitus Treatments – Have you tried all of these? http://Tinnitusdx.com/blog/Tinnitus-relief/top-17-Tinnitus-treatments-have-you-tried-all-of-these/. Accessed 2 May 13.

Types of Tinnitus, http://www.Tinnitus123.com/types-of-Tinnitus/, accessed 28 February 13.

Treatment Information, http://www.ata.org/for-patients/treatment#Biofeedback, accessed 1 March 13.

Virage Sante. http://www.viragesante.com/en/. Accessed 9 June 13.

What is acupressure? http://www.acupressure.com/, accessed 1 March 13.

What is Acupuncture, http://www.whatisacupuncture.net/, accessed 1 March 13.

What is Cochlear Hydrops? http://www.wisegeek.com/what-is-cochlear-hydrops.htm, accessed 12 August 13.

What is reflexology? http://www.reflexology-research.com/whatis.htm. Accessed 4 June 13.

What is Pseudotumor Cerebri Syndrome? http://www.wisegeek.com/what-is-pseudotumor-cerebri-syndrome.htm, accessed 24 August 13.

Made in the USA
San Bernardino, CA
19 January 2019